Exploring the Home Health Care Experience:

A Guide to Transitioning Your Career Path

Kathy Quan RN BSN PHN

ISBN 978-1517320027
ISBN 151732002X

Medicare rules and regulations change often. Always seek counsel from the experts in your agency or refer to the regulating agencies such as Medicare

Advanced Praise for *Exploring the Home Health Care Experience….*

Want to learn what it is *really* like to work in home health care? Your first step should be to get two copies of this book—one for your bedside table and the other to keep in your car. It should be required reading!!
Donna Carol Maheady, EdD, ARNP, Founder of http:// ExceptionalNurse.com
http://exceptionalnurse.blogspot.com/

Kathy Quan RN BSN PHN does it again. Another book chock full of information, real world experience and resources. Professionally written and based on experience, Kathy shares valuable tools for those interested in home health. Trust me, from someone with no home health experience, I now feel more equipped to work in this type of role!
Elizabeth Scala, MSN/MBA, RN, bestselling author of 'Nursing from Within', http://elizabethscala.com/

Home care is an expanding market that requires sharp, clinically competent professionals who can work independently and think outside the box. *Exploring the Home Health Care Experience: A Guide to Transitioning Your Career Path written* by Kathy Quan is an important resource that nurses can use as they move beyond the bedside into the dynamic world of Home Health Care.

This *'must read book'* will help you understand the nuances that come with this arena and illustrates the important role nurses play in ensuring patients are safe, understand how to manage their chronic healthcare needs as well as have the tools they need to have successful outcomes.

This book is an excellent primer for all healthcare professionals responsible for transitioning patients to home as well as those who provide and oversee the care delivered in the patient's home.
Anne Llewellyn, RN-BC, MS, BHSA, CCM, CRRN
Nurse Advocate
http://nurseadvocate5.blogspot.com

Acknowledgements

I would like to thank all of my social network nursing contacts for your continued support of my efforts to help nurses find their way in this profession and to shine.

I also want to say a special **Thank You** to:
Anne Llewellyn, RN-BC, MS, BHSA, CCM, CRRN (http:// nurseadvocate5.blogspot.com/) for her editorial assistance. She brought a new set of eyes to this book and asked the questions I would expect of anyone exploring this field for the first time.

And finally to all the professionals I have worked with and known through my 35 plus years in the field of home health and hospice. You inspire me and provide me with so much valuable information and experience to share here and on my websites: HomeHealth101.com and Housecalls-online.com.

Dedication

This year has been a busy one with weddings and the birth of my first (blood) grandchild. She arrived 3 weeks early and threw us all off our game! You all kept me going and made me stick to deadlines to get this book finished. You inspire me to help others be better health care professionals and make this a better world for all of us. Thank you so much Mom, Jo, Tim, Amy & Eric, Rob & Yoli, Ally, Sophia, and Becky & Wes! Love you all!

Happy Reading!

TABLE OF CONTENTS

Foreword

This book is designed to help nurses and other health care professionals make the transition from other fields to home health care. This publication can be used alone, or as an accompaniment to, *Exploring the Home Health Care Experience,* a Power Point presentation by Kathy Quan RN BSN PHN. Both are available at KathyQuan.com and Homehealth101.com.

Private duty (shift) home care is often confused with skilled intermittent home health care and the terms are many times used interchangeably. In fact, they are two very different entities. This book and the optional Power Point presentation will exclusively pertain **to <u>intermittent skilled</u>** home care. However we will touch upon the private duty aspect for purposes of information, resources and differentiation.

As we progress from a sick model of health care delivery to a wellness model of health care in the U.S., home health will continue to be one of the fastest growing areas of health care for a variety of reasons including cost effectiveness, and better and faster healing options. Home health care is a vital option to the continuum of are and reducing hospital readmissions.

Home health is one of the most rewarding fields, especially for those who enjoy spending one-on-one time with patients, caregivers and family members. It affords nurses, therapists (PTs, OTs, STs), home health aides and social workers more quality time to spend teaching patients and caregivers how to assume responsibility for their own health status. As in any other field of health care, a typical day can be very routine and quiet (*don't say that out loud*) or it can become extremely intense, challenging and even chaotic.

Home health care can be one of the most challenging fields both physically and emotionally. Creativity, flexibility and innovative abilities are just a few of the most important characteristics home health professionals MUST posses.

At one time, home health nursing was considered to be somewhat of a "second class" career option. Home health nurses weren't actually considered to be "real nurses." The same could be said for home health therapists and social workers. Over time with the advent of better and more mobile technology, along with changes in admission criteria and reimbursement in both the acute care settings and home health, this opinion has changed.

Patients are now discharged home from the hospital and post acute settings much sicker than ever before and home health care is quite often a preferred option for aftercare. Home health care is also much more frequently used in lieu of hospitalization when feasible. Home health nurses have learned to manage some of the most complex cases at home with IVs, chemotherapy, home dialysis, ventilators, chest tubes and Pleurex draining systems, wound drainage pumps, and many other complex treatment modalities.

Home health therapists engage in much more complex rehab programs in the home setting than ever before. In many ways this meets the needs of the patient better and more effectively because the patient is learning skills and tips in his own environment and not in a rehabilitation or skilled nursing facility setting that may have no similarity to the patient's home and environment.

Social workers in home care face an abundance of challenges in providing counseling and resources to help patients regain and/or maintain their independence in their own homes as long as possible, or find suitable placement options. They have to be able to get passed patients' inane fear that they are there to wreak havoc in their lives. Social workers must convince patients and their families and caregivers that they are indeed on their side and will work to make life easier with the goal to maintain independence for as long as possible by helping them attain the skills and resources to make changes when necessary.

Learning something new often feels like you are moving backwards from the expert to the novice. Transitioning to home health care is no exception, but it can be one of the most rewarding career changes you can make! Explore your options and see if this isn't your best next move.

Introduction to Home Health Care

Today more health care professionals are exploring home health care as a career focus or for additional income as a per diem or part time position. Home health care can offer the flexibility that can meet many different employment needs.

Back in the day (70's and 80's) there was a requirement that nurses had to be BSN prepared and have a PHN (Public Health Nurse) certification. That requirement began to slide and by the 90's, only those seeking management career paths had to have this certification. With continued rapid growth in the field in recent years, a PHN is rare today although a public health 5th semester option is still available in many BSN programs.

Without the PHN, the significance is that more nurses come to home health care with limited exposure. They may have had one clinical rotation. It's something they more likely fall into through the recommendation of friends and acquaintances rather than aspire to from a rotation in the course of the education.

In practice and in theory, home health care affords the practitioner the opportunity to use all of their training, expertise and education to work with patients one-on-one without constant interruptions from another patient or co-worker on the unit or in the facility. However, this is not without challenges and exasperating moments. Patients and caregivers can be distracted by a variety of situations in the home as well such as missing their favorite television program, outside visitors coming and going, and phone calls. Setting limits and parameters for the home health visit time is critical to success for all disciplines, but must be sensitive to the patient's desires. Sometimes it is necessary to schedule visits around that favorite program, or to reschedule when unexpected visitors arrive.

Home care professionals often have to be a Jack-of-All-Trades, but be confident that no one ever expects you to go into a home alone and unprepared. One of the best advantages we have today is the availability of information and technology. Between the Internet and sites like You Tube, you can almost always find pictures and videos demonstrating procedures and technology. Be open and honest if something is new or you are uncomfortable. DO NO HARM.

Home health care indeed is NOT for everyone. As we will explore in this book, it takes a certain skill and personality to succeed in this realm. It can be difficult, it can be lonely, it can be scary to be without a colleague nearby, but it can be the most rewarding experience all at the same time. If your sole goal for your home health career is to work "*banker's hour and have weekends off*," this may not really work out for you. A strong dedication to your patients is required here. Yes, there are some great perks, but there can be struggles as well.

Home health under a pay-per-visit plan can afford professionals an opportunity to make a significant salary; however quality patient care must always be the goal. Those with strong assessment skills, efficient and effective teaching skills, and great organization skills can be very successful in this field and have significant financial gains. Those who wish to skimp on quality care and outcomes just to make a six-figure living should really consider another field.

There are basics you will need to understand. *NOTE: Some readers have been well versed in part of this information and it will be boring and something to skip over. For others, I hope it will be useful and informative. Background information in my opinion helps to build a foundation and leads to a better understanding how and why things work as they do. To me this is an essential part of enjoying and surviving home health care.*

To be frank and honest, there is such an overwhelming amount of paperwork, and it will never ever go away. Understanding the necessity doesn't make it any less cumbersome, but it does make it logical and hopefully easier to manage. As you begin to understand the purpose, you should begin to understand how to answer the OASIS questions, why they are necessary, and why each form is essential to justify the care your patient needs and deserves. We will cover the OASIS in detail.

Beyond the paperwork, it's important to understand a couple of concepts and decide whether they are things you can work with. The first is that you will be working with patients in their own home or place of residence such as a residential care facility for the elderly (RCFE) such as a small 4-6 bed board & care home or a larger assisted living facility. These are essentially considered the patient's "home" as well. This means you will be *a guest in that home*. You will be directing the implementation of the plan of care for that patient, but there's a distinct difference from directing care in a clinic, facility or hospital where it's more or less "your home ground." This time it's in the patient's home.

You can still be assertive and forceful, but you MUST be respectful of their home, their belongings, their animals, and their family members, loved ones and their caregivers. In other words, you can't bulldoze into the home and make demands to get rid of things, move things around and take complete charge.

Every effort you make for the safety, well-being and good of the patient has to be done with tact and respect for their home and possessions. You will have to make many small steps in the process and respect that things may be right back where they were when you return. This can be very difficult for some, and frustrating to all of us.

In a hospital, you have the authority to re-arrange the furniture, put the personal possessions in a closet, and turn off the TV. In their home, you need to ask first and provide education and information to support your suggestions. Often you can garner cooperation if you start with the changes most necessary and consider them to be temporary until the home health care is completed. If patient's have the sense that they will be able to change back in a short time, they regain the control although they are relinquishing it temporarily. Compromise is a key point.

The second consideration is that like most any other realm of health care, you will have to discharge the patient; and that may be sooner than you would like. Discharge planning begins with the start of care and continues with each and every visit as you set and accomplish goals and outcomes.

You will get attached to some of your patients. That's human nature to bond with some. But you have to let them go. Your job is to teach them how to improve their health status, take responsibility for it and move towards improved outcomes. And then you have to let them fly on their own. Of course, if they need you again, you will be there for them.

If you can't let them go, then as supervisors have told me, and I have told many a professional I have supervised, *you need to take them home with you*! That usually helps with the separation anxiety. And please, don't be tempted to give them your personal contact information!

Home health is about teaching patients and their families and care givers how to rehabilitate from an illness or injury; how to prevent complications and recurrence; and how to improve their overall health status and outcomes.
The model is to help patients become responsible for their own care and health status. It's not just about sick care, although you will provide some in the process.

Patients come home from the hospital sicker. Other times, the physician in lieu of hospitalization orders home care. Home health care is intermittent. It's not shift care, and it's not acute care. Our job is to go in and assess, make a plan of care, instruct and evaluate the response, make changes if necessary or continue on. (Sound familiar? It's the Nursing Process in action.) The patient is the center of the plan of care and must buy into it or we have to find some other option.

Newcomers to home health often have the inclination to do everything for the patient because that's most often how it works in the hospital setting. There's no time to educate patients; you just have to do it. Hopefully they will pick up on how to do it themselves by watching you. In home care, the patient or able and willing caregiver is expected to assume responsibility for the care as soon as possible under the watchful assessment, evaluation and supervision skills of the nurse or therapist.

This can be one of the most difficult parts of transitioning to home health care for professionals. For instance, ICU nurses make great home care nurses because they have sharp assessment skills and although they don't diagnose, they can pick up on symptoms that may be overlooked by nurses from less acute care backgrounds. But they also have some of the hardest times letting go and letting patients do for themselves because they provide such intense bedside care.

This can be especially true when IVs are involved. I have witnessed ICU nurses driving themselves crazy worrying over leaving a patient alone in their home with an IV running. What if it infiltrates? What if the cassette infuses faster than it should or needs changing? They're on the phone with patients every 2-3 hours, or spending sleepless nights worrying themselves into exhaustion and even illness.

You do your best at educating the patient and caregivers in all aspects of the care required. You place the agency's 24/7 access phone number near the phone. And then you have to take a leap of faith. Pumps will alarm if there's problem. On-call professionals can troubleshoot over the phone or send out a nurse if absolutely necessary. And patients/ caregivers really do learn to care for themselves and all of the equipment. They may develop some unconventional means for doing so, but with guidance and supervision, they will survive and thrive.

A therapist has to eventually leave the patient alone with his DME and know that they can manage. Hoyer lifts are perhaps one of the scariest devices ever, but patients and caregivers really do master their safe use. And hip and knee replacement patients do recover and rehabilitate to move on with their lives.

Another issue that can seemingly overwhelm newcomers to home health is that not every patient comes with tasks and instructions from the physician or hospital. Sometimes our job is to go and observe and be the eyes and ears for the physician. Check out the home for safety problems. See how they manage their medications. What kinds of food do they have in their home. (They're on a low sodium diet and they have a freezer full of frozen meals, and a pantry full of canned foods all high in sodium.)

Some times you just have to go and complete the OASIS questions. Perhaps this will provide clues. And then you have to get them to SHOW you how they do things. Have them TELL you what each medication is for. And you'll be surprised at how many will tell you their heart meds for instance, are vitamins or just something the doctor gave them to make them "feel better or stronger." You'll discover clutter and throw rugs that create safety hazards. You'll find no rhyme or reason to their medications and bottles and bottles of expired pills.

And when you're all done with your assessment, you may still have to discuss your goals and plans with a group of seasoned home care professionals. You will work alone out there, but you have an entire team of professionals to consult and plan with. And the physician has oversight of the care.

Sometimes there will be no skilled need and you won't admit the patient. But you'll still be the eyes and ears of the physician in that home and can report to him/her your findings. This can be valuable information for the physician, and help to instill his trust in you as a home health professional. You can provide the patient with valuable resources and information and if a need arises, be the point of contact he makes for his future care.

Learn to be a sponge. Pick the brains of everyone around you. Some tips will work well and others won't. You will find a niche of your own and a groove. Give yourself time. Be flexible. Ask for help, but don't whine and be overly needy. You are a professional. Have confidence in your skills. You won't have ever done it all, so ask for help with new things.

Learn to use resources. The Internet is full of the, but know how to find reliable resources, and don't believe something just because it's on the Internet. Improvise. You won't always have sterile saline. Know how to make it on the fly. Learn the strengths and weaknesses of your colleagues and don't be afraid to ask for assistance.

Enjoy your freedoms, but don't procrastinate. The best time management is about managing your own procrastination, Be organized and prioritize. Be flexible, but not a doormat. For instance, gas is expensive. You can't accommodate everyone and crisscross all over town everyday.

There are rules and guidelines for home health that affect business decisions, operations and reimbursement. If the agency doesn't get paid, you may not either. Other rules affect how you will conduct business. NEVER give out your cell or home phone number or other personal contact information!! (Block the ID each time you make a call.) Protect these always, and if inadvertently they are discovered, make sure the patient or caregiver knows they must call through the agency for everyone's protection and best interest. Be HIPAA aware, don't discuss the patient with his well-meaning neighbors. Always be alert to your surroundings and don't go in if you sense it's not safe. A supervisor or colleague is always a phone call away. Do No Harm! If you've never done something or are uncomfortable, ask for assistance. Learn to enjoy your new role.

CHAPTER ONE: Why Choose Home Health?

Health care offers many superb opportunities to individuals with the passion for caring for others and making a difference in people's lives. For each of us, the places our career leads us will involve very personal reasons and choices.

Just like any other option, home health care won't be the best choice for all health care professionals. I know I could never have survived the constant adrenalin rush and frenetic pace of the ER. ICU got too technical for me before I had a chance to really give it a try. I didn't enjoy making snap decisions when I didn't have the time to carefully assess a situation.

For me, teaching patients and their caregivers how to make a difference and improve their health status and outcomes was a primary interest. I found it very frustrating to try to do much teaching in the hospital setting. Frequent interruptions for other issues; sometimes important and too many times trivial, just made me crazy. I knew from my public health rotation in nursing school that home health care is where I could find satisfaction and success. To prepare for that eventuality I worked in med/surg for a couple of years right out of school.

My unit was a mish-mash of many acute and chronic diseases and challenges. At that time, patient stays were much longer, and we had a fair share of revolving door patients who would go home for short periods and then return because no one was helping them adapt and learn to care for themselves at home.

Today, patients don't have that option, and in fact, are often are pushed out the door before they even settle in for one night. Studies have repeatedly shown that patients do better in their own home. They are certainly less likely to catch a nosocomial infection, and they are more likely to be encouraged to fare for themselves instead of depending on others.

Nothing quite equals sleeping in your own bed, eating your own food choices, and setting your own rules. But patients have to have the tools and help to manage their care at home. They need a support system and they need education.

Over half of the population in the US is considered to be health care illiterate. This means that they have no idea how to get health care, what is expected of them, and how to follow through once they do get some help. Further, they don't know enough to know what kinds of questions to ask to help them get the information they need.

For example, you may be very surprised to find out that some members of your own family wouldn't know they have to refill a prescription, much less know how to do it. For people who have never experienced a long term or chronic illness, their only experience with prescriptions has most likely been limited to taking antibiotics for a few days. And at that they may not have taken the medications as directed. Many people stop taking medications as soon as they feel better. The job of the antibiotic isn't finished until the last pill is being coursed through the body. We have to educate people to complete the course of any medication, and if it's to be ongoing they have to call to refill it in advance of running out.

Whether or not the patient has been hospitalized, anyone with an illness is not at his or her best. Add symptoms such as pain, nausea, vomiting, anxiety, anorexia or constipation and you have a decreased ability to concentrate and /or cope. Mix in some wounds or incisions, or surgical repairs of fractures and you have even more difficulties in learning and coping.

Discharge a patient home in 2-3 days and he may feel abandoned and could panic. This was often the reason for the revolving door patients returning in the old days. Today it's still true and emergency rooms are overcrowded with patients who don't know how to care for themselves. And they most likely will still not get sufficient information and answers they need to keep them from returning to the ER.

Hospitals have been mandated to reduce readmissions due to the unnecessary costs incurred because patients haven't been sufficiently educated in self-care to ward off symptoms requiring medical attention, or the knowledge to notify their PCP instead of rushing to the ER. One of the ways this can be accomplished is to involve home health agencies that are also under the gun to reduce hospital readmissions and have the opportunity to work with patients on a one-to-one basis.

When the discharge planners and case managers can offer patients follow up care and teaching at home the next day, patients will often have a much better mindset for facing their new health challenges. And if the doctor can refer to home health from his office, many patients can avoid hospitalization all together and contain costs that way.

Home health nurses have to have a broad range of skills from medication and diet teaching to inserting a Foley catheter or finding a vein in a dehydrated little old lady for lab work or IV therapy. They have to know how to manage traches and sometimes ventilators, G-tubes, wound vacs, home dialysis, and chemotherapy. Then they have to instruct the patient or caregiver to maintain the patency and integrity of these, and how to avoid infection or complications.

Therapists also need to have a broad range of skills and expertise and be able to work independently.

All home health professionals need to have the latest applications for their smart phones or laptops and they need to know how and where to find information and resources for their patients. They need to be jack-of-all trades and know how to improvise and find answers when something is new to them.

You won't have another nurse, therapist or medical resident down the hall to drag in and ask for help or an opinion. But you will have a whole support system of colleagues and supervisors who are a phone call away. The important thing is to always remember to DO NO HARM. Turn to your own support system of colleagues and mentors to keep you and the patients safe. And then be a sponge and learn every new trick, technique and resource.

Nursing is a lifelong learning experience and home health care is one of the best examples of this. This applies equally to all other home heath professionals.

WHY IS HOME HEALTH A FAST GROWING FIELD?

Based on data from the U.S. Dept. of Labor Bureau of Labor Statistics, the primary focus of nursing and patient care in general is switching from the bedside and hospitals to home health care. Currently 25% of the population in the USA is over 55. The fastest growing segment is over 80 and of that, those who are 90+ make up the largest group. The U.S. Census Bureau estimates the population of 90years+ being 10% of the population by 2050; and 1 in 5 Americans will be 65 or older by 2030.

As this trend continues, many more nurses will be needed to meet the needs of the aging population along with therapists and social services. A specialty in geriatrics and the needs of the elderly will be needed as well. Many of the elderly suffer from chronic diseases and other factors that make them homebound, meaning it takes a TAXING EFFORT to leave home and a significant recovery time after doing so. Consequently this limits access to the health care system. To meet the needs of this population, home care visits will be necessary for follow up education and care after having a qualifying face-to-face visit with their PCP.

The elderly are prone to falls. According to the Centers for Disease Control and Prevention (CDC) Millions of older people —those 65 and older—fall each year. In fact, one out of three older people fall each year. Unfortunately, less than half tell their doctor. Falling once doubles the chances of falling again.

Today 1 in 8 older Americans have Alzheimer's disease; 1 in 4 has Diabetes that can contribute to falling. According to the U.S. Census Bureau, in 2014, 46.2 million Americans were 65 or older. Their median income was less than $25,000 per year.

The skyrocketing costs of health care have also forced a lot of changes in the health care delivery system. Where once patients were admitted to a hospital for tests and teaching purposes which could last a week or more, today much of that is accomplished as an outpatient and the teaching done either in a clinic setting or in the patient's own home.

For example, twenty-five years ago when a patient was suspected to have diabetes they were hospitalized for tests and diagnostics. Then once started on a regimen, they remained hospitalized until their mediations and diet fairly regulated their blood glucose levels. If blood sugars got out of control, they would be re-hospitalized to stabilize them.

Today, in rare instances this may be the case. Most patients receive brief education from their physician's office and are given a prescription for their meds and some literature to read.

Unfortunately, that aforementioned healthcare illiteracy can quickly come into play and you'll have a confused patient trying desperately to make sense of it all while drowning in information he doesn't understand enough to even question. If the physician was thinking proactively, he may have referred the patient to a diabetic educator, or to a home health agency for diabetic teaching. Home health nurses often deal with diabetic education.

The high cost of health care also forces patients who qualified for admission to be discharged from hospitals long before they have recovered. They may go home while still receiving a course of IV antibiotics. They may have suffered a stroke and are in need of extensive rehabilitative therapy from Physical Therapy, Occupational Therapy and ST or Speech and Language Therapists. In lieu of extended inpatient care, they may be sent home to recover with assistance from a home health agency.

In the past home health care patients were primarily elderly and on Medicare. A young patient with private insurance was rare. Now private insurance companies and MediCaid provide coverage for home health care to a much younger population in lieu of more expensive options such as hospitalization. Much of the care needed today can be provided in the home for patients of all ages.

With a rapidly aging population, a physician may need the assistance of the home health care nurse or therapist to assess an elderly patient or couple for their ability to safely remain in their own home. They may need some education about their acute or chronic illnesses and medication management. A PT may be needed for a home safety evaluation, transfer training or a home exercise plan to build strength and improve balance.

An OT might be indicated for energy conservation techniques as well as ADL (activities of daily living) and IADL (instrumental) activities of daily living) tips and tricks. ADLs include eating, transfer/ambulation, bathing, dressing, toileting (continence), and grooming. And IADLs include such things as shopping, cooking, laundry, housekeeping, managing finances, using a telephone, driving or using public transportation.

They might also need an MSW (medical social worker) for community resources and for short term and long term care planning. When the elderly parents live far away from their adult children, home health can step in and help teach the parents how to remain in independent in their own homes for as long as possible; or help them transition into a more appropriate level of care. The MSW can often assist with applications for MediCaid/

MediCal, getting long term care insurance in place to cover private duty care or placement, and procuring caregivers or placement if needed.

The home health staff become the eyes and ears of the physician and provides an insight into the reality of the home situation. Perhaps that sweet lady with CHF is non-compliant with elevating her lower extremities because she has no place to do so. She can't afford a reclining chair and is embarrassed to tell the doctor. She has no ottoman or footstool and her coffee table won't work in a pinch. Her only option would be to lie down in bed, but that makes her feel like an invalid and cause stiffness from her arthritis to exacerbate. She keeps telling the doctor that she tries to elevate her lower extremities several times everyday. But when he learns this is not actually possible, he has to make changes to the plan of care.

Postoperative care for joint replacements is another area where patients are sent home soon after surgery to recover with home health care. Skilled nursing care can include managing post-op wound care; monitoring anticoagulant therapy and instructing in bleeding precautions along with other post operative care. This can include teaching patients or caregivers how to give lovenox or heparin sub-q injections.

Physical and Occupational therapy would provide home safety instruction and a home exercise program for joint replacement after care.

IV hydration for pregnant women with hyperemesis can be done in the home setting. Other chronic illnesses such as Multiple Sclerosis (MS) or Rheumatoid Arthritis (RA) are often treated with IV medications that can be infused in the home setting and even in the workplace by home health nurses when insurance companies cooperate. Long-term antibiotic therapy is another option seen in home care for treatment of acute illness such as osteomyelitis.

Teaching patients and caregivers to manage sub-q injections such as lovenox, heparin, various insulin, RA drugs, interferon, etc., can be done in the comfort of the patient's home by home health nurses. In addition, the home health nurse monitors the effectiveness of the medication or possible side effects and reports back to the physician. Other important and preventative health education can be provided as well.

The Palliative Care Mandate

Palliative care was mandated to be included in home health care programs by 2014. This can affect patients of all ages with acute or chronic illnesses involving symptoms out of control. These include symptoms such as pain, nausea and vomiting, constipation and diarrhea, anxiety brought on by the illness itself or treatments such as chemotherapy or radiation.

Palliative care encompasses a wide range of diseases beyond cancer such as congestive heart failure, kidney failure, COPD and other chronic lung diseases, MS, and severe forms of arthritis. In some cases, some of these patients may be hospice appropriate, but not ready to accept hospice as yet and palliation of systems becomes more essential. Still others are not considered terminal and may recover with some intensive help with their symptoms and find improved quality to their lives.

Medicare is exploring a Palliative Choice Model for hospice to improve patient care options. Participants have been chosen and a demonstration program will begin in late 2015.

INTERMITTENT VS. PRIVATE DUTY HOME HEALTH CARE

For all intents and purposes this book is primarily about intermittent skilled home health care as opposed to private duty home care that may or may not be skilled care. The difference is vast, but the two are often limped into one category. We will cover this in depth throughout the book, but for now this is a brief discussion of the differences.

Intermittent skilled care requires a licensed health care professional such as a nurse or therapist to perform and /or to teach the patient or caregiver to perform the skilled task and then assess the progress at varying intervals until the care is no longer needed or the patient/caregiver are proficient in the care. This includes skilled care such as wound care, post-op care, rehab or home exercise therapy post injury (fall/fracture or surgical repair or replacement) or illness (CVA), dietary and medication instruction, disease management (i.e. diabetes, CHF, COPD). As long as the skilled care is needed and the patient is making measurable gains a social worker, dietician and home health aide may also provide care.

In private duty the skilled care is usually for long-term cases such as patients on ventilators, or any other need for 8-12 hour shifts up to 24/7 care. Their care is often mixed with custodial care. Custodial care is unskilled and can be performed by a licensed or unlicensed person depending upon the preference of the patient. Assistance with ADLs such as bathing, dressing, grooming, ambulation, toileting, feeding are a large part of the care provided in addition to other tasks such as laundry, light housekeeping, shopping, errands and transportation for the consumer. If administering medications or performing invasive procedures such as tracheostomy care or g-tube care is involved, a skilled nurse must perform this level of care.

Intermittent home health care service is sometimes referred to as "the visiting nurse" or "the visiting therapist." It involves visits from skilled health care professionals such as nurses, therapists, social workers, home health aides, and dietitians who have been trained to proved care in the patient's home when the patient meets specific criteria for care. [We will discuss this later on in Chapter Two.]

The visits are typically 45 minutes to an hour long and the skilled professional provides care and instruction to the patient, family members, and any other caregivers. These visits are spaced out (intermittently) according to the need over several days or weeks and continue as long as there is a skilled need, the patient continues to make measurable gains and meet criteria, a valid plan of care with a physician's oversight is in effect, and a valid source (with authorization as needed) of reimbursement for the visits exists.

In rare instances, the patient may wish to continue visits and pay privately for them if he or she no longer meets criteria for reimbursement from Medicare, Medicaid or Private Insurance. This is typically for therapy visits after the patient has met their maximum rehab potential, but desires to continue the therapy to coach them along. It's expensive, so it's rare, but can be done.

Private duty home health care is care provided in the home, but under different circumstances. The care does not have to be skilled. It can be custodial in nature and quite often is. Unlicensed caregivers such as companions and homemakers can provide private duty home care. This level of care is an *out of pocket expense* and not reimbursed by health insurance, MediCaid or Medicare. If the consumer so chooses, a licensed nurse (RN or LPN/LVN) can provide the care, but this is a matter of personal choice and does not make the care skilled.

Most agencies require a four-hour minimum each day for private duty care. The frequency is determined by the need and the financial ability of the consumer. It could be a one-time need or a daily occurrence, or any combination in between.

Private duty care can also be shift care provided by registered or practical nurses for patients requiring a combination of skilled and custodial care on an on-going basis. This may or may not be reimbursed (in whole or in part) by health insurances and MediCaid. It is never covered under Medicare. This care can be respite care for a parent or other family member who usually provides the care, it can be care provided while the family member sleeps or works outside the home or in addition to the care of the family member depending upon the need and the financial or reimbursement coverage.

HOME HEALTH IS NOT LOW-TECH ANYMORE

Home health care got a bad rap many years ago for being very low tech. Home health nurses were looked down upon by the nursing community and some went so far as to infer that home health nurses weren't really nurses. I would challenge that on any given day, back then or now.

Today, there is nothing low-tech about home health care. Even on a routine visit just to change a Foley catheter, the nurse will most likely record her visit documentation on a laptop, tablet or hand held computer device. She may use a digital thermometer to take the patient's temperature in her ear or by swiping her forehead. Then she may take a digital photograph of the funky looking urine with her smartphone to text or email to the physician for his orders for lab and or treatment options.

Laptops, tablets, hand held computers, and smartphones are common sights in any health care setting. Glucometers, finger-stick testing for PT/INR, pulse oximeters, oxygen concentrator and ventilators, wound vacs, various IV and sub-q pumps, etc., are just a few of the more high tech options that have become part of the everyday life of home health professionals and their patients.

Therapists have options with tools such as ultrasound and mini whirlpool devices. New designs and modifications to these and other devices provide for a constant need for in-services to keep staff up to date on the latest state-of-the-art equipment and upgrades.

As the needs of the population change, technology will meet the challenge to provide many more modalities in the home.

Florence Nightingale's Influence on Home Health Nursing

We don't often associate Florence Nightingale with home health nursing. We see her on the battlefield in the Crimean War saving soldiers with hand washing, hygiene and sanitation. But Flo also worked in schools, sick houses and workhouses taking care of patients and teaching them and their families and caregivers how to incorporate these same universal precautions and infection control techniques in these settings and throughout their lives.

Today, we continue to instruct in these techniques in all avenues of health care. In home care we encounter all sorts of hygiene, sanitation and infection control issues!! While we have to remember we are invited guests and this is *their home*, we also have to provide them with the information to help them understand how to improve their well-being and outcomes by making changes to their home settings and habits. This takes patience and tact!

CHAPTER TWO: Criteria for Home Health Care

One of the most important concepts to understand is: *meeting criteria for home health care*. This is perhaps the most essential part of the **Conditions of Participation** and being eligible for reimbursement for the care provided. You can't admit a patient just because you have an order from a physician to do so.

As we discussed in Chapter One, the care <u>must</u> be skilled; not custodial, and not just an evaluation. We briefly touched on this subject and some of the other factors that help the patient meet criteria. In this chapter we will expand on this to cover all of the criteria.

The 3 primary criteria are:

- Homebound
- Skilled Need
- Physician's Orders for Care and care plan oversight

1. HOMEBOUND

Perhaps one of the most complicated and misunderstood concepts is homebound status. To qualify for Medicare coverage for home health care, the patient MUST be homebound. (Private insurance and Medicaid usually follow Medicare's regulations for home health guidelines, but in some instances they are not as rigid with this criteria. Be sure to check this status for each patient under your care.)

The theory behind this requirement is that if the patient is not homebound, he can seek medical care elsewhere such as at a clinic or outpatient physical therapy. Therefore to be reimbursed for caring for patients at home, they must meet the homebound criteria.

One of the things that confuse this issue is that patients seeking treatments such as dialysis or chemotherapy are quite often considered homebound despite leaving home 2-3 times a week for these treatments.

Homebound is not black or white. It isn't set in stone and must be applied to each individual case. Sometimes, despite the best efforts to define homebound, the homebound status may be fuzzy or unclear. You must discuss this with your administrative staff, and in these situations, careful documentation is essential. It would be expected that the episode of care would be short.

For purposes of discussion in this book, we will consider homebound to be necessary for all home health care patients unless otherwise stated.

Homebound is not always a permanent condition, but must be in effect during the entire length of stay (episode) on home health care. Once the patient is able to freely leave his home, home health care must come to an end.

One of the most important facts to remember is that just because the patient cannot drive or doesn't have a car does NOT make them homebound. Housebound yes; but not necessarily homebound.

Homebound means that it takes a taxing effort for the patient to leave home, and because of this he only does so on infrequent occasions. This must be documented and it is most easily done by describing the effect of leaving home such as exhaustion upon return, increased weakness afterwards, having to nap upon return home, an increase in shortness of breath, etc. Be sure to give specifics and measurements such as after returning from church, it took him 3 hours to recover and not be short of breath at rest.

If the patient now requires the assistance of a device or another person to ambulate safely with or without a device (walker, cane, crutches), this too can be a reason they are homebound. The frequency of leaving home and how it affects the patient will further help you decide the homebound status.

After an accident, acute illness or post surgery the patient may be homebound due to pain with movement, weakness, unsteady gait, poor endurance etc. that causes it to be a taxing effort to leave home.

For many more options to document homebound status by condition/disease see: http://homehealth101.com/ homebound_status/homebound_statements/ diagnosis_related_homebound/

If the patient is bed bound, then of course, the homebound criterion is met. However, but it must be consistently documented that the patient remains bed bound, as this too could be a temporary circumstance.

The OASIS tools will help to define and justify the level of homebound status with the selection of appropriate answers that provide clues to the patient's functional status and limitations. These limitations need to be consistently documented throughout the episode of care.

2. SKILLED NEED

The second criterion is having a **skilled need**. This means the care is medically necessary and requires the education and skill of a nurse or therapist to perform and oversee. The nurse or therapist may then teach the patient or caregiver to perform this skill. Once the patient or caregiver demonstrates the ability to perform the task(s), the nurse and or therapist will oversee the patient's progress by assessing 2-3 times a week, making changes to the plan of care as indicated, and instructing in the revised plan of care.

Therapy typically sees the patent 2-3 times a week for 2-3 weeks to instruct in a home exercise program (HEP) designed to rehabilitate or strengthen the patient after an episode of an illness, injury or surgery. The HEP will be revised as the patient attains measurable goals, or fails to meet them. When the patient has met all goals or proves to be unable to meet them, the therapy must end. The therapist may also provide the patient with instructions for an ongoing self-guided program to maintain his strength and balance.

Home safety inspection and instruction is part of all home health nursing and therapy. It's a skilled need to ensure that safety risks are explored and instruction provided and measures taken to prevent them. Falls are the biggest safety risk and must be assessed. Physical and occupational therapists can assess for DME needed as well as placement of grab bars. The OT can assess for energy conservation techniques to improve the patient's endurance and reduce related safety risks. It can be the only skilled need, but the plan of care will be a short one.

The nurse may encounter patients who need a variety of levels of care. They may need an IV started and instruction in how to manage the equipment to provide multiple doses, flush lines and understand how to contact the agency for troubleshooting problems and complications. There may be blood levels (peaks and troughs) to draw and results to report to the physician for possible changes in treatment.

Or the nurse may be performing wound care to an incision or decubs or skin tears. She may be instructing the patient or caregiver in how to change the dressings, what signs and symptoms to report to the MD, and how to improve healing with enhanced nutrition, position changes, etc. She may decrease her visit frequency when the patient or caregiver is competent just to assess for healing or complications.

Nurses may provide instruction in disease management such as diabetes (diet, medications, blood testing, exercise, etc.) or CHF (salt management, daily weights, medication adjustments, and signs and symptoms to report).

These are skills the nurse or therapist went to school to learn. They can be taught to a patient or caregiver, but the assessment of the process and outcomes and what needs to be done next is something the skilled professional continues to provide.

When the patient or caregiver becomes proficient with the care, the follow up care can be directed back to the physician and the home health care should end. Therefore, the nurse may not see a wound completely heal, or the therapist may turn the patient over to outpatient therapy long before he meets his maximum rehab potential. But the job has been well done when the patient can carry on and not return to the hospital with reoccurrence or complications from unfinished instruction, treatment or assessment.

3. PHYSICIAN ORDERS and CARE PLAN OVERSIGHT

The third component of the criterion is a physician's order and oversight of the care plan and any changes made throughout the episode(s) of care.

The patient care plan is collaboration between all of the home health team members and the patient bases on the skilled needs and the physician's orders. The orders must be authorized and signed by a physician willing to continue to provide oversight.

The hospitalist may have made the original referral to home health care, but the patient's physician (primary care or specialist) must be willing to oversee and sign orders for the agency to provide home health care.

At the present time only an MD, podiatrist, or DO will be signing the orders. It is hoped that in the future legislators will change this so that NPs and PAs (nurse practitioners and physician assistants) will be able to sign orders and provide the oversight as well. This would be especially helpful in locations for example where there is a shortage of physicians and these professionals provide much of the primary care. This is a good example of how Medicare being a federal plan takes precedence over state regulations. For non-Medicare certified agencies, the NP or PA can sign orders for care, but not for the Medicare-certified agency. Home Care associations have been advocating to change this for quite some time. Under hospice, the NP can sign orders.

BREAKING NEWS: As we go to press (Oct. 2015) so to speak, Congress is considering a bill to allow NP's to certify patients for home health care. The Home Health Care Planning Improvement Act is a measure aiming to permit nurse practitioners, clinical nurse specialists and certified nurse midwives to sign off on home health care

plans and authorize Medicare patients for home health benefits. For more information: http:// homehealthcarenews.com/2015/10/bill-giving-nps-more-home-health-power-gains-momentum/

ALL care must have a physician's order. Any changes must be approved, and the supplemental order signed, by the physician. This includes things such as simple modifications to wound care. For instance, if you had to use 4X4's instead of mepilex because you ran out, you need to get a temporary order for that day because you need to document exactly what you did. Everything that changes the Plan of Care must have a signature from the physician. (Next time you'll be sure you have adequate supplies!)

If the patient has several physicians, it is best to have the primary physician to agree to oversee and sign all orders, but s/he may want the orders sent to the specialist physician as well just to keep him/her apprised of the changes.

As of 2011, per the Affordable Care Act, if the patient was not hospitalized within 14 days prior to the start of home care, then there must be a **Face-to-Face visit with a physician 90 days prior to the start of care or within the first 30 days of care**.

An NP or Clinical Nurse Specialist collaborating with the physician can make the Face-to-Face visit, but the physician still has to sign the certification of homebound status and skilled need until that law changes. The physician must sign a form attesting to this visit and indicate the reasons s/he is ordering home health care based on the findings at that face-to-face visit. And certifies the physician has current knowledge of the patient's health status. This is required for Medicare coverage and reimbursement.

These rules were tweaked again in 2015 to make it easier to document the skilled need and homebound status in the narrative portion. Going forward, I expect the rules to be changed frequently. The new rules put the burden on the home health agency to get the background documentation that supports the MD decision. CMS is trying to make adjustments for the complicated process and allowances for face-to-face documentation errors.

CONDITIONS OF PARTICIPATION

In simple terms, CMS (Center for Medicare & Medicaid Services) along with the U.S. Congress established a set of rules and regulations (Conditions of Participation) for Medicare Certified home health agencies, often referred to as the COPs.

 Each state may also have a set of regulations, but the Federal rules always supersede state and local regulations. Congress updates these regulations at least annually and when finalized they are published in the Federal Register and CMS sends out updates. Many of the annual rules involve financial issues and reimbursement and then other rules are altered to help meet the criteria.

The Medicare Benefit Policy Manual -- Chapter 7 defines intermittent home health care and lists the rules and regulations (CoPs) that Medicare Certified agencies must follow. The most updated copy will list the recent changes in RED along with the implementation date. This policy is also referred to as the HIM 11 and can be downloaded in .pdf from CMS.gov at https://www.cms.gov/Regulations-and-Guidance/.../bp102c07.pdf

Newcomers to Home Health Care should familiarize themselves with these rules to get a basic understanding of what is allowed and what is expected. Each discipline's role is outlined along with policies for supervision such as the supervision of the Home Health Aide (HHA) every 14 calendar days. And LPN/LVNs can work in home health care as long as they are supervised by an RN and adhere to their state's scope of practice. The RN delegates tasks for the LPN/LVN to perform and report back to the RN.

POLICIES and PROCEDURE MANUALS

Each agency will have their own P&P manual and employees are expected to read and follow these procedures and policies. CMS makes routine unannounced survey visits to provide oversight of Medicare Certified Agencies. They make home visits with clinical staff to deem adherence to such things as policies and procedures, bag technique, trunk policies, sharps hauling permits, as well as patient specific care. Be sure to locate and utilize your P&P manual, especially if a surveyor is making a visit with you.

CHAPTER THREE: Qualities for Home Health Professionals

Home health care presents some very different demands that are not part of other health care fields. The care is provided in the patient's home or sometimes in RCFE facilities such as board care homes or assisted living facilities. Skilled nursing facilities provide nursing care and therefor don't utilize the home health care benefit as it would be a duplication of services. Each of these settings presents certain challenges to meet the rules and expectations. These can change on a dime when the players change such as a new Director of Patient Care Services at a facility, or a new caregiver in the home setting.

It is our responsibility to provide the care that the patient needs and to work within the boundaries and dynamics of the setting. Wherever the patient resides, this is his home and we need to be mindful of this and respectful of his home. Although we have an important purpose in being there, we are guests.

It is not our focus to come in and bulldoze our way around making changes according to what we consider to be important. Rather we need to adapt to the patient and his environment and do what we can to make it safe and effective. This is not always easy.

As you will see in home health care, you might have visits in any given day that take you from the ghetto to the most opulent neighborhoods and you'll be working with patients who have little to nothing all the way to those who have no financial ceiling. In a similar fashion you may see a full gamut of education, abilities and desire to improve their health status. Their expectations of your role and their own in the plan of care may differ dramatically as well. Many will completely surprise you.

You will be thrown in the middle of family dynamics the likes of which you will never want to be part of again. There will be patients who have no family or friends and you will need to keep your professional distance and not want to adopt each and every one of them. In short, you will find a new appreciation for your own challenges and situations.

First and foremost you need to be **experienced** in your field (nursing, therapy, social work) and **confident** in your abilities and skills. You also need to remember that you have a support system of supervisors and colleagues to call upon when you are stumped. You have to be comfortable asking for help. This is not the time to try to be all things to a patient or to bluff your way through a procedure you've never seen before. Expect to feel like you know nothing and that you have transitioned from an experienced professional to a novice. This will quickly fade as you learn your new role and gain confidence.

You need to be **organized** and **efficient**. You will have a full schedule of patients to see in a day, and the paperwork (even if it's point of care on a laptop) can be overwhelming!!

Along with that, you do need to be **flexible** and able to change your day around at any given time if a patient's needs require it.

Home health professionals who are highly organized will fare well in this arena. Those who are not, will struggle and can become lost and overwhelmed very quickly. Time management skills and organizational skills can be learned and should be a priority for anyone transitioning to this field.

There will be times when you will have to use your **imagination** and be **innovative**. (*Necessity is the mother of invention.*) If you don't have enough wound dressings, what can you do? You may be an hour's drive from your office. **Improvise**. Use some paper toweling to reinforce on the outside of your base dressings to make them more absorbent and go further.

If you don't have another sterile catheter, can you do something to re-use the one the cat contaminated when he flew into your sterile field out of nowhere? Yes, hot soapy water can cleanse the catheter, and you can boil it for a few minutes to truly sanitize it.

Care in the home is considered clean, not sterile. Unless you're dealing with IV lines or care that must be sterile, clean technique is the routine. This is the patient's environment and he has immunities to it. Tomorrow you will get the proper supplies and replace things you had to make do with today. It's not a perfect solution, but in a pinch it will work.

You need to be **assertive**, but not aggressive and be able to tell the difference.. Your role is to teach patients and caregivers to provide the care. Give them the knowledge to prevent future problems and to know what and when to report to the physician. Build trust and a rapport with your patients and they will respect you and listen to you. If you try to change too much too quickly you'll put them on the defensive they won't hear what you say, and certainly won't be cooperative and compliant.

Set Limits with patients and families/caregivers who get caught up in the one-on-one attention and think you are at their beck and call. Do NOT give them your cell phone number! Explain that communication needs to be tracked and must go through the office. Skilled staff are available 24/7 to answer their questions and needs. Discuss appropriate use of after hours calls for urgent issues only. Encourage them to write down their questions or concerns so that they can be discussed at scheduled visits. Communicate with other disciplines and manage the Plan of Care.

Tact is an essential quality. You aren't there to judge anyone. Your role is to help them learn a better way to achieve an improved health status. Always remember this is their home and their lifestyle. You must respect their right to it. You may not makes these choices, but they have. Calmly, you will want to make suggestions that can help them move in the right direction if their choices are adversely affecting their outcomes and health status.

If something is a safety hazard such as smoking while using oxygen, you must be firm and explain the danger it presents to others as well as the patient. Most times you'll find they have never even considered that all of the tenants in the whole apartment building could end up homeless and/or injured just because they don't care if they blow themselves up. Given this new perspective, they might try harder to be careful.

Throw rugs are a danger to anyone, but many people see them as something that makes their home warmer, nicer, and some have sentimental value. Suggest ways to tack them down, hang them for decoration, or place them outside of major walkways such as under the dining table.

You must always **be professional** and remember that you are a representative and ambassador of your agency. You need to be well groomed, wear clean clothes or uniforms and **closed toe**

shoes. Your hair and fingernails should not be barriers to providing clean and safe care.

Be mindful of scents. Perfumes are not necessary. If you smoke, be aware that it permeates your hair and clothing. Foods such as garlic and onions can give you offensive breath.

Scrubs and good sturdy sneakers or professional shoes work best. They can be sanitized and the shoes not worn into your own home. Some of the places you will go are not the cleanest and you don't want to wear your best clothes and shoes in to some of these homes.

In facilities, always introduce yourself and make your presence known at each visit. Let them know when you leave. Sign logs and ask to see their paperwork so that all the rules are being met. **Communicate!**

Effective Oral and written communication is an essential skill. You will be the doctor's eye and ears and need to keep him/her informed of the situation. You may need to communicate with relatives who live out of town and help them make informed decisions. You must be mindful of HIPAA at all times and avoid violations.

If you are the case manager, you need to **lead** the home health team and organize and execute the plain of care. The paperwork in home health is endless and you will need to understand what is required and expected and how to embrace the situation to ensure reimbursement as well as meeting the needs of the patient. Listening is an important part of communication so you need to be a good listener.

You need to **be patient, compassionate, empathetic** and **have a passion** for providing care to patients in challenging environments. Your safety and welfare will always be the concern of your agency. If it's not a safe place to go you need to communicate that to your superiors. You need to be acutely aware of your surroundings at all times and be proactive.

Home health care is one of the most rewarding fields where you can truly work with patients and their families and caregivers one-on-one to improve their health status and outcomes.

However, it's not the place for everyone. This is especially true for those who don't like to work alone, can't self-direct, or lack confidence in their skills.

CHAPTER FOUR: The Typical Day

Productivity expectations will vary from agency to agency especially when geographic issues come in to play. More rural areas will have lower productivity expectations due to extended travel time. Those who see a majority of their patients in one or two RCFE's may have a higher productivity ex[ectation.

As the new kid on the block, your patient load will be lower initially. You will spend a certain amount of time shadowing and working with one or more preceptors to learn the ropes. Be a sponge, learn as many tips and tricks as you can. Get a feel for the culture of the agency, the doctors you get referrals from, and the kinds of patients you will typically see.

As you develop your own caseload, you may find that you have a specific geographic area, or you may cover a wide space depending on your expertise, your status as full time, part time, per diem, etc.

Some agencies practice true case management where you follow your own patients and delegate them out if you have too many for the day. Other agencies will make patient assignments. You may see some of the same patients over and over, and others will be patients most often seen by someone else. Make sure you know what all is expected from you for these visits such as OASIS forms, re-certifications of service, orders for more care after this visit, etc.

Typically you'll start out slow with a few established patients. You may spend part of your time with a mentor, preceptor or staff educator who will help assist you with the paper work or point of care process after you complete your visits for the day. You may have a couple of new starts of care interspersed as well to help you build your own caseload and learn the paperwork.

PLAN YOUR DAY

Plan your day around geographic locations as best you can. This will conserve gasoline and wear and tear on you. Sometimes this will be impossible because the task at hand requires a specific time such as teaching a new diabetic about fasting blood sugars and morning insulin. Try to schedule the worst cases as early as possible. These might be tasks you dislike, patients who are difficult, dysfunctional families, etc. Get these over with and move on with your day without them weighing you down all day long.

Have a clear plan of your goals for each patient. Read previous notes to review progress made and to set your goals. Have a clear understanding of what else may be expected of you for this visit beyond the patient care such as a report for your private insurance coordinator to obtain continued authorization, or an update phone call to a relative. And have a good idea of the expected measurable gains to look for and document.

Call each patient to remind him or her of your visit today. Ask if they need any supplies, if you're providing any, and give any pre-visit instructions such as pre-medicating for pain or holding a medication until the blood is drawn.

Try not to give patients a specific time except perhaps for your first visit of the day. Give them a 2-4 hour window and explain that you cannot predict any closer due to unexpected delays with other patients, traffic, etc. You can offer to call them when you're on your way to their home if that helps.

Make an effort to work around their special needs such as naps or must-see TV programs, but remind them that you have several patients to see and your time as well as gasoline is a premium these days.

Once you become established, you'll find a routine. A typical day could involve 6-8 revisits to established patients who require varying degrees of care. Or if you have new starts of care, they typically count as 2-3 revisits and therefore you should have fewer revisits that day.

You might have 2-3 patients who are fairly new to your service and are still being educated in the steps for their own care. There will always be someone who resists taking full responsibility for his or her care. Sometimes this is a person who lives alone and has no willing and able caregiver to assist her. Perhaps she is post op with a wound dehiscence that needs irrigation and packing which she is not able to visualize nor accomplish without a third hand. This visit will take a little longer as you try to find ways for the patient to use mirrors and improvise for that third hand.

Perhaps you'll have a patient who is making measurable gains in transfers and ambulating very short distances with his walker. He is 2 weeks post op from hip surgery (ORIF), but is very frightened of falling again and doesn't trust his caregiver to assist him. The tasks of building patient's confidence in the caregiver and ensuring that home safety standards are met are taking a little longer than usual. This visit will be a little more challenging than some of your others.

You may have 2-3 visits that are very routine. You'll be observing the patient or caregiver demonstrating the care you've instructed in and assessing for changes as the patient improves. These visits can take 30-45 minutes and present little to no challenges -- carry on.

However, be prepared, these can sometimes present surprises as patients and caregivers improvise on their own with unsafe or non-standard practices. Are they pushing the patient to ambulate further than you instructed? Did they decide to skip an important step in the wound care that they deemed redundant or unnecessary? Back up, explain why this is unsafe, and review the correct way to do things.

Remember, the reason there is a skilled need is that these are lay people who don't have the level of education you have. Always be prepared for the unexpected, and don't assume your directions are being followed to the T. Even if they are, there can be complications. Despite everyone's best practice, a wound can become infected. Complete compliance with a new medication regime can hit hiccups or have an adverse response.

As you become more established, plan on being interrupted throughout your day with calls from your office to address calls from patients, family members and physicians. Learn to expect the unexpected. Just as in the hospital setting, the best-laid plans will be vulnerable to patient issues.

Foley catheters will fall out or become obstructed, IV pumps or lines will need attention, dressings become soiled or fall off, and patients will fall. Some of these you'll be able to handle over the phone. Some you'll be able to delegate to another nurse or therapist with the help of the office, and some will mean an added visit or two for your day. And perhaps pushing off a more stable patient until tomorrow. It's the story of your life as a health care practitioner to prioritize and re-prioritize. This is just exactly why you can't promise specific times to your patients.

PAPERWORK

Try not to work on paperwork during the visits except to jot down measurements or vital signs. Laptops can be even more of a distraction. Be present with the patient and give your undivided attention. The most difficult times will be when completing the OASIS forms, but as you become familiar, you should be able to complete these later as well.

After each visit you should complete the necessary paperwork so that things are fresh in your mind. Some practitioners stay in the home to accomplish this. Regulations require that the patient or caregiver sign your notes to verify you made the visit and finishing the note is highly recommended.

Point of service laptop programs can require that you complete the previous visit note in order to open this one and get a patient signature. If you didn't complete the note for your last visit, you may not be able to open this note snd get that signature. Staying in the home affords you the opportunity to re-check something or to perform a task you forgot. You may also need to contact the physician to report on findings or to obtain new orders for care.

This time also gives the patient or caregiver a few minutes to think of questions or concerns they forgot to bring up earlier. On the other hand, some patients or caregivers will get a little uncomfortable and want you to move on. So move to your car. If you need to go back in, you're still right there.

The important thing is to complete the visit by finishing the paperwork before moving on to the next patient. Sometimes this is not feasible but try to make it the norm and not the exception.

Procrastinating with your paperwork can cut into your family time or build up and get you way behind. Your own paycheck will be dependent on turning in paperwork timely. Conditions of Participation dictate that paperwork be filed in, or synced from your laptop to, the chart within set time frames. OASIS paperwork has to be reviewed and transmitted to Medicare in short set time frames. Get your paperwork turned in in a timely manner and you'll not have that monkey on your back.

Phone calls to physicians, delivering blood samples to the laboratory, interdisciplinary consultations, are just some examples of tasks that are related to a specific patient and become part of that specific visit. These should <u>all</u> be documented in that visit's notes. Who you spoke to, where and what time you left the blood sample, and any expected follow up.

Agencies that pay on a per-visit basis usually expect that the time involved is included in the per-visit rate. On occasion if the time spent is excessive, there might be additional compensation made, but this needs to be discussed with your supervisor prior to or right after the occurrence.

There is no perfect employee payment option for home health care. You will have to have faith that it all comes out in the wash so to speak. Some days will be better, and some days you'll be spending all sorts of what can seem like extra-unpaid time.

This can be true even if you are paid hourly. Your supervisor isn't likely to approve a lot of overtime. Nor will you be allowed to drop your productivity frequently because you have a lot of labs to draw in a week. Discuss this with your supervisor ahead of time and try to come to the best compromise.

Home health also affords you some freedoms you won't find in other jobs. It will be important to recall how you were able to see your child receive an award at school midday by taking an hour break in your day. These occasions will wash with times you have to spend on extra patient related items.

CHAPTER FIVE: Why So Much Paperwork?!

Before discussing the types of paperwork required in home health, it's important to understand why there is so much and why it's not going to go away. We'll go in to detail on the OASIS (Outcome and Assessment Information Set) and prospective pay in a later chapter.

One of the reasons for the ever-increasing amount of paperwork is that there has been a long history of Medicare fraud and abuse in home health care. This exacerbated in the 1980's and was rampant in the 1990's extending into the early 2000's. Home health agencies sprung up almost over night across the country simply because it was rumored to be a quick and easy way to make money for owners and administrators.

Home health care was reimbursed on a fee-for-service basis, meaning they paid by the visit. The more visits made, the more money they made. Many of these owners/administrators who abused the system with unnecessary visits or even charging for visits that weren't actually made, have paid heavy fines. Additionally, some have served, or are currently serving, prison terms for their actions.

Congress and Medicare (CMS - the Centers for Medicare and MediCaid Services) have taken multiple actions over the past 3 decades to reverse this trend and have drastically reduced the fraud and abuse in home health.

The Balanced Budget Act of 1997, and amended by the Omnibus Consolidated and Emergency Supplemental Appropriations Act (OCESAA) of 1999 set in place requirements for the development and implementation of a prospective payment system (PPS) for Medicare home health services to curb costs and reduce fraud and abuse.

CMS surveyed agencies in a rapid-fire manner and discovered patients weren't homebound. Too often visits documented weren't actually made. There was no skilled need or medical necessity documented. If there was a genuine need at one time, the goals had long since been met and visits were continuing for no clear reason. In dramatic, almost witch-hunt fashion, agency after agency was shut down after failing a CMS survey. Even the best, quality agencies feared being surveyed and possibly having their doors closed.

Once the way was cleared for quality agencies to continue providing legitimate and good care, the plans were put in place to help ensure honest and ethical practices would be the trend. One way has been to increase the amount of paperwork to ensure compliance and raise the bar in collecting data and reporting measurable statistics for every patient.

The OASIS data collection process and Prospective Pay by episode of care were born. This payment reformation was mandated originally by the Medicare Reform Act of 1997 and renewed again in 2003. Congress deemed it necessary to collect data to prove that home health care actually improved outcomes. The Affordable Care Act again addressed the OASIS and adjustments have been made to the data sets and criteria.

OASIS data is collected on all non-maternity patients 18 years of age and older. The data set items encompass a holistic view of the patient including psych-social demographics, environmental, social support system, clinical health status, and functional status attributes of each patient. Pertinent diagnoses that explain the skilled need and medical necessity are coded with appropriate ICD9 codes to further provide data to help determine the episode payment. By October 1, 2015, home health agencies had to update to the use of ICD10 codes as an industry standard.

The data is collected by the nurses and therapists and subsequently transmitted to CMS at specific time points from the beginning of an episode of care to the discharge from care.

Reimbursement by Medicare is now based on a set flat rate per episode of illness. Additional tweaks are made to the flat rate fee depending on case-mix data for certain diagnoses and conditions. This is accomplished through specific information and answers to questions in the OASIS data set. Instead of a fee-for-service basis, agencies are paid an all-inclusive lump sum to care for the Medicare patients for 60-day intervals.

Private insurance and MediCaid reimbursement sources continue to pay on a negotiated rate for fee-for-service basis. Most require prior authorization for visits and some actually utilize some or all of the OASIS data to review for skilled need, medical necessity and outcomes.

The burden of the OASIS paperwork falls mainly to the nurses and therapists. In addition to providing excellent quality care, home health professionals have to utilize the OASIS forms to prove that the care is medically indicated and warranted, and that they have set and either met or been unable to meet measurable goals and why. This information gets reported to Medicare and is shared on the Internet with consumers. On the CMS website, consumers and practitioners alike can compare one home health agency with another based on how well they meet multiple criteria with their patents.

For instance, if you are looking for the best agency to help rehabilitate your mother after total hip surgery, you can compare several agencies on the site for their ability to meet goals necessary to recovery from hip surgery. You can visit the Home Health Compare site: http://www.medicare.gov/homehealthcompare/

The data for the comparisons is pulled from the OASIS data that is collected at specific points throughout the episode of care. Again, the OASIS process will be discussed in greater detail in a later chapter.

CMS now also reports data on physicians, hospitals, dialysis centers, and nursing homes for consumers based on other data collection processes to compare when making health care decisions. This is expected to continue and expand.

Documentation is a major part of health care in this country, and in home health it has always been a burden. Even with the Paperwork Reduction Act, paperwork is a huge consideration in home care.

As a health care practitioner, you're not going to escape the burden of documentation. For home health professionals it has always been a part of their daily process. Completion of the documentation at the conclusion of the visit is the best possible scenario for accuracy and timeliness while it's fresh in your mind.

Measurable Goals

Your documentation provides evidence of skilled need along with measurable goals and your patient's progress. You will also have to continually provide evidence of the homebound status. (See Homehealth101.com for sample homebound statements : http://homehealth101.com/homebound_status/ homebound_statements/diagnosis_related_homebound/)

You should not use the words "evaluate" or "monitor". You are a health care professional making a **skilled assessment**. Based on your skilled assessment, you and the patient will make a plan of care and discuss it with the physician. You will then direct the plan of care.

You will determine the success of the plan by re-assessing. As needed, you will modify the plan of care and again ensure the buy-in from the patient and the approval from the physician.

You will in fact, practice the Nursing Process. The nursing process uses "evaluation" as part of the terminology, but CMS is touchy on this matter. Therefore it's important to use terminology to depict a skilled process that cannot be confused with an unskilled level of care.

If you utilize any form of the word "evaluate" it should be differentiated as a "skilled evaluation" or assessment of the situation.

Measurable goals may be lofty or expect very minimal progress depending upon the situation. The plan of care will be unique to each patient. You will use standard statements to convey these goals, but you will also need to adjust them to fit each situation. You will need to document the success or failure to meet the goals and provide information as to why the goals were met or why not.

Terms like "more," "more and more", and "more and more and more," may imply progress but they are not measurable. You will need to cite specifics such as percentages, exact or approximate distances, size and shape of wounds, etc. Photographs can be used to help document especially when words are not capable of describing the full extent of the circumstances.

For example, a patient with severe and multiple contractures can best be represented by a photograph. Wounds should always be photographed at various stages of healing to ensure clear understanding of the status.

In home health care you will expect to see improvement in status over time. In re-evaluating and resetting goals, you will need to update information and revise your goals. The ultimate goal is to help the patient become and stay as independent as possible and to **reduce hospital re-admissions.**

Reimbursement from Medicare, or other source, for the care you provide depends on the documentation. *Remember, if you don't chart it, you didn't do it.* Beyond that, what did you do? What is the response or outcome? What needs to be done next? If you don't document completely, you leave the agency vulnerable should the case be reviewed by the payment source.

A Few Tips to Improve Documentation

- Be sure to state facts and not opinions
- Use the patient's own statements- Quote him: *patient stated,"blah blah."*
- Answer the questions: <u>Who, What, When, Where, How and Why</u>?
- Have a goal for each visit. State it
- Show your work--- what did you do? Teach, demonstrate, assess, re-educate, assess return demonstrations?
- What was the effect or outcome?
- Was your goal for this visit met?
- What is your new goal for the next visit?
- Did you communicate with the physician, other disciplines, caregivers, etc? And what was the result?
- What discharge planning did you provide in this visit?

See Sample Documentation on HomeHealth101.com <u>http:// homehealth101.com/documentation_examples/sample-documentetion.html</u>

CHAPTER SIX: Safety Issues in Home Care

Organizational skills are imperative to home health professionals. You need to pre-plan for possibilities, expect the unexpected, and be proactive at all times.

One of the most important points to remember always is that YOUR safety comes first. A request for care may initially come from a patient or the patient's family or friends, but the patient's physician must give the order to make an assessment. The physician must certify that s/he has had a Face-to-Face encounter with that patient specific to the needs of the home health care. However, the physician most likely has never visited the patient's home. So it cannot be assumed the referring physician has any knowledge of the safety of the home geographically or environmentally. The home health professionals must always be alert to unsafe situations and conditions and discuss them immediately with an administrator level person if there are dangers or hazards.

In every city there are known neighborhoods that are less than ideal, and some that are downright dangerous. However, that being said, you cannot always judge the safety by the cover. In some volatile gang areas, the visiting nurse or therapist may be the best-protected person in the vicinity. Knowing that you are there to help so-and-so's grandmother could elevate you to "king or queen for the day" status. They may instruct someone to sit and watch over your car and or to escort you. However, not everyone may feel comfortable driving, parking and walking through specific neighborhoods even with a personal escort. This will be something you will need to review with your supervisor and other team members. Alternative plans may need to be implemented or the case referred back to the physician if it is truly an unsafe situation.

Always double-check an address over the phone before you make a visit to a patient you haven't seen before. And ask whether it's a house, condo or apartment and if there are any tricks or tips to finding the place. You'll also want to inquire if there are dogs present and ask that they be secured somewhere. Never make eye contact with a dog or trust that it won't bite you!

Never park in the patient's driveway unless you have been instructed to do so. It would be a good idea to inquire as to nearby parking restrictions at your pre-visit phone call. You won't be given a free pass to violate posted restrictions just because you're the home health worker. Park in well-lit and accessible public areas only and take note of your surroundings before you leave your car. Lock your car!

Make note of the surroundings as you walk to the patient's home. Have your purse or other personal items secured in the trunk of your car before you arrive at the patient's home. Only take in the items you need to have. They should fit into your bag of equipment or an additional disposable bag. Pockets can hold small items. Keep your keys handy and your cell phone in your pocket. You might want to carry pepper spray and/or an animal deterrent, but be sure you know how to use them correctly so as not to harm yourself or any innocent person or animal.

Don't be texting or talking on your phone as you approach the home. Be alert. Always pay attention to your gut feeling. If it doesn't seem safe, don't go. And don't let your guard down even though you've been there many times.

If it seems iffy, TRUST YOUR GUT and call your office and ask them to call you in a few minutes to check on you and arrange to call them again after you return to your car. Some nurses have called the police department and asked for an escort for weekend and after hours visits, or to have the officer patrol the area while in the home and then contacted the officer when they had returned to their car.

The vast majority of your visits will be safe and secure, but always be alert to a situation that might present challenges.

Encountering an unexpected dog can be a problem. Never trust that they "never bother anyone." And never make direct eye contact with an animal.

UNIFORMS VS STREET CLOTHES

This is an age-old battle. Uniforms and scrubs are much more professional and may actually command more respect for you from your patients, family and friends as well as those hanging about in the neighborhood. In some areas they might invite trouble thinking you may have drugs with you. Your agency will have worked through this issue and be best at advising employees what to wear.

One of the best arguments for wearing uniforms or scrubs is personal infection control. You will be in and out of homes all day long. Some will be spotless and others cluttered and filthy. You'll be dealing with a multitude of bodily fluids and treatment situations. Uniforms and scrubs can easily be sanitized in the washer and even removed in the mudroom before entering your own home. The same can be said for shoes. Do you really want to wear your best shoes into some of the homes you'll frequent? Keep your nice clothes and accessories for outside of work. Protect yourself and your family from uninvited germs and debris. Always wear safe, comfortable closed-toe shoes.

A lab coat or vest can be quite useful. Pockets are required for this job. For instance, you may not want to take your bag in to certain homes and yet you need some basic equipment with you. Pockets are ideal. So are large zip lock Baggies which are disposable.

YOUR CAR - YOUR HOME AND OFFICE AWAY FROM HOME

You will want to be sure to keep your car in tiptop shape. The gas tank should always be kept above 1/2 full. Change the oil and fluids as recommended and make sure tires, belts, windshield wipers and hoses are changed as needed.

For your taxes you'll need records of these expenses so keep track and anticipate the next servicing to avoid being caught off guard. You will also need careful records of the mileage travelled for work. Keep a notebook in your glove box.

You will need to make sure you have non-perishable snack food and water at all times. Keep them cool and fresh. You'll never know when your day will run long or the weather or other factors keep you from getting home. Inclement weather will be a nemesis, but a manageable one if you are prepared.

Always have an umbrella in the car. An extra sweater or sweatshirt and pair of socks stashed will be a welcome find on many an occasion. Even an extra set of scrubs and undergarments can be handy too.

Have a flashlight handy and a supply of fresh batteries. In colder climates a large candle in an old tin coffee can be a great emergency light and heat source. And you may want to carry an empty tin can in case you need an emergency toilet in a storm as well. An old blanket and pillow could come in handy on many an occasion as well.

If you use handwritten charts you will need a safe place to store patient charts and extra forms. A plastic file box can house extra forms and paperwork. You can store patient charts in there as well if you have room. Otherwise a second box is ideal or even a small plastic tub with a lid.

YOUR TRUNK

You will need to keep your bag and extra supplies in your car. Your trunk is the best choice for these. *Be sure to keep the clean items separate from the dirty items*. Never transport medications. Dispose of unused or expired medications in the patient's home per your agency policy. You will need to have a sharps container and a hauling permit from your local government authority. The sharps is a prime example of the dirty supply area to separate from new wound supplies, catheters, etc.

Rotate your supplies so that you always have new items in your car stock. If you find you aren't using items, return them to your supervisor for permission to return to the supply room.

Be mindful of expiration dates, and try not to expose your stock to extreme temperature changes due to weather conditions.

Large rubber or plastic bins can work well to keep the supplies organized and separated. Make sure the area is contained and separate from all personal items and don't use the bins to hold groceries or other non-work related items.

On the other hand, keep all of your equipment stored so that your family and friends don't access it. Never have supplies lying around in plain sight in your car. If syringes are visible, someone might think you also have medications and this can become a dangerous situation. Keep a shoebox or other small container inside your car if you're going to keep supplies for today handy. Make sure you can't see into it.

Your purse and other personal items should be locked in your trunk, or hidden inside your car before you make your first visit. These items should never be accessed in view of where you will park and leave the car unattended.

Keep a dollar or two, or your lunch or snack money in the glove box for convenience or in your pocket.

YOUR BAG

All home health professionals should have some sort of bag to carry their equipment such as stethoscopes, thermometers, sphygmomanometer, gloves, hand soap, paper towels, tape measures, calipers, pens, note pad, etc. This should be a separate bag from your paper chart, laptop, iPad or other point-of-service device.

BAG TECHNIQUE

When you enter a home you should also have a clean barrier such as a chux or newspaper. Place this barrier down on a solid surface (NEVER on the floor or patient's bed) and put your bag(s) on top of it. If there isn't any place to set it down, ask the caregiver to bring a kitchen chair or TV table. And request this be present for all home health care visits.

- Your hand soap and paper toweling should be in an outer pocket of your bag. Wash and dry your hands before proceeding. Ask to use the bathroom sink if at all possible. Hand sanitizer and supplies to clean your equipment should also be in an outer pocket.

- Next find another clean barrier such as more paper toweling to set down your equipment. Reach into your bag and take out each piece you will need for the visit and place them on the new barrier.

- **DO NOT re-enter your bag unless you rewash your hands first!**

- Clean all equipment and then wash your hands before returning it to your bag at the END of your visit.

- Complete your documentation and be sure you answer all questions the patient or caregiver think of while you take a few minutes to complete your documentation.

- Dispose of all trash in a small bag and secure. (Double-bag any soiled dressings or other contaminated trash.) You will place this in the outside trash after you leave the home or direct the caregiver to do so. And instruct them to wash their hands after handling it.

- Use hand sanitizer (which is also in the outside pocket of your bag or in your pocket) after disposing of the trash. DO NOT take the trash with you.

- Place any dirty items in your designated TRUNK area, and proceed to the next location.

RESTROOMS

Except in an absolute emergency, you should never use the bathroom at your patient's home. Find a clean public restroom. Make scheduled stops. Libraries, Starbucks, fast food and department stores are usually great locations to memorize and save on your GPS. Many gas stations, convenience, grocery and drug stores may have good accommodations as well. You'll learn where the best spots are. Pay attention to your preceptors. They will have a list already.

LUNCH

Pack a lunch if you can, as your day will be full of interruptions. Nutritious foods are best from home, and expensive and inconvenient to find on the road. If you can't pack a whole lunch then be sure to pack some nutritious snacks. Keep water with you at all times. Beware of letting water in plastic bottles get hot in your car. Sources say they can leach chemicals into the water. Metal canteens are a good alternative. A small ice chest or soft-sided cooler is a necessity. Reusable ice packs can be frozen over night for the next day's use. It's helpful to have a few on hand in case you forget. A thermos with hot soup or broth can make your day if it's wet and cold outside.

CELL PHONE

Your cell phone is an essential tool. Aside from communication, it can be your camera, as well as your access to the Internet for information and resources. Keep it charged. Have a car charger on hand or an optional back up battery or charger. And keep it secure.

DO NOT provide your patients or their family members with your cell number. Insist they contact you through your office. Even if others on staff give their numbers out, explain that it is NOT your policy to do so. Block your number when you make calls to patients and family members. (Do this as well if you use a landline phone from your home.) If they inadvertently obtain your number, instruct them NOT to use it. You won't be answering it at night or on your days off.

Your privacy is important to you and your family. You don't want to be called by patients or caregivers at 2 AM if you're not on call. And you don't want to be responsible for messages left that you never received. Your agency will have numbers to be reached 24/7.

Instruct and prepare patients and caregivers in how to contact the agency, how to use the after hours system, and what to do if there is an issue with the phones or someone doesn't call them back.

Keep your cell phone in working condition. If it's damaged or lost, and it's the only way your agency can contact you, you MUST obtain another phone ASAP! In the event you are on-call let the after hours service, along with your supervisor, know how to contact you and/or make arrangements to call them every hour until you can get an alternate phone arranged.

If your agency doesn't provide or reimburse for cell phones, check with your tax advisor for deductions for your phone, as having phone access is a requirement of the job.

You might consider having an extra cell phone for work to keep it separate from your personal phone. Be sure to check your plan to ensure you have the most economical one possible. You don't want to have huge bill at the end of the cycle! Be proactive.

Remember any patient information MUST be encrypted (use a medical record number) and safeguarded on devices and on paper at all times. Photos should be transferred to the computers in your office and deleted from your phones according to your agency policy. Patient information should be transcribed and removed from your devices at the end of each day.

CHAPTER SEVEN: What is This OASIS?

Paperwork in home health care is one of the biggest complaints heard from staff. It is often far more time consuming compared the paperwork in hospitals, clinics, facilities and professional offices combined. However, when you understand the purpose and begin to work with the system, it does get easier! There will be a learning curve, but after you get past that, and settle in to a routine, you will love your home care career.

BACKGROUND

The OASIS (**O**utcome and **AS**sessment **I**nformation **S**et) can be one of the most daunting sets of paperwork ever known to health care workers. And this was designed in the early years of paperwork reduction!

It is a lengthy document and often filled with redundant questions. If you aren't consistent in how you answer these, an error report will be generated for the OASIS guru in your agency to investigate at a later date. Don't worry, you'll become proficient at it and eventually master the process.

Per Medicare, OASIS is a group of data elements that:

1. "Represent core items of a comprehensive assessment for an adult home care patient; and
2. Form the basis for measuring patient outcomes for purposes of outcome-based quality improvement (OBQI)." [http://www.cms.gov/Medicare/Quality-Initiatives-Patient-Assessment-Instruments/OASIS/Background.html]

In a jointly funded project between CMS and the Robert Wood Johnson Foundation, the data items were derived and have been tweaked ever since. The purpose of the OASIS is to monitor home health care and evaluate the outcomes. It stemmed from a Congressional act (The Balanced Budget Act of 1997) specifically aimed at reducing costs and Medicare Fraud that was rampant at the time.

The OASIS data set has gone through many changes since it's origin in 2000 and likely will continue to do so in order to meet the ever changing needs of Medicare recipients, and comply with the transparency edicts of the Affordable Care Act and future legislation processes moving forward. The OASIS data collection and transmission process and policies have been changed to meet (and exceed) security and HIPAA privacy needs and will continue to evolve along those lines.

The OASIS is designed to assess and evaluate the patient's needs and outcomes during the course of stay (an episode of care) on home health. The data from these outcomes is also used to compare and benchmark with other agencies. The benchmark findings are reported quarterly on the CMS Home Health Compare website for consumers to use when electing a home health agency.

The OASIS data is also used to provide the basis for Quality Assurance and Performance Improvement (outcome quality based) processes at the agency level. Feedback is derived from the data and sent back to the agency for study and improvement. The details of all of this are available on the CMS.gov website and from your own OASIS and Quality department within your agency.

The purpose of this chapter is to present the basic OASIS process to help the novice become acquainted with the process and hopefully resolve some of the overwhelmed feelings associated with the OASIS. For more in-depth study of the OASIS process, the CMS.gov website provides a massive amount of information for home health professionals.

The OASIS is time consuming. Every agency is well aware of the time impact the OASIS has on every OASIS visit. The admission to home health care or Start of Care (SOC) is usually the most impacted visit due to the OASIS length in addition to the actual care and teaching necessary at that visit.

Whether the agency pays per visit, hourly or by straight salary, accommodations are almost always in place to ensure that you are compensated for your time, and productivity numbers are adjusted to account for OASIS visits in your daily schedule.

That being said, for those new to home care, obviously this process will have a learning curve and like with any new job you need to understand that eventually you will become more efficient at this process. It all comes out in the wash eventually. If there is no difference in compensation or productivity, perhaps you need to reconsider your options.

OASIS BASICS

There are 5 main components to the OASIS process. They are:

1. Start of Care (SOC)
2. Recertification ("Recert")
3. Transfer
4. Resumption
5. Discharge

SOC OASIS

An Episode of Care begins with the SOC and continues for 60 calendar days. At SOC you will assess the <u>clinical, functional and social issues</u> and document them on the OASIS. If the patient meets criteria for home health care, **the SOC OASIS** stands to justify the need and eligibility. Remember, you must have a skilled need for an RN or Therapist (PT or ST) to establish care. The patient must be Homebound, and you have to get the approval for your POC from the ordering physician.

This is NOT a document to hand to the patient or caregiver and ask them to answer the questions! This is the professional health care worker's comprehensive, patient-specific evaluation and assessment of the patient's clinical, functional and social status.

You MUST check the most appropriate box as applicable to the *situation at this moment*. A numerical value is assigned to the boxes and only numerical data can be transmitted to CMS. Your comments and explanations cannot be used. You must make decisions based on the information given and asked for.

There are also **Skip Patterns**. For instance, if a question is not applicable, move on. Be sure to follow the patterns and directions to skip to the next designated question.

As you assess for ADLs and IADLs, ask the patient to actually perform the tasks such as unbuttoning/buttoning his shirt. Some items you will be able to assess from what has already happened. Such as, did the patient ambulate from his chair with his walker and oxygen tubing to let you in at the front door? How stable is he in doing this as he returns to his chair? Is he SOB despite the O2? Is he alone? Or is there a caregiver? Is he clean and well groomed? Is his shirt buttoned all wrong? Is the TV blaring and he keeps asking you to repeat yourself? Or is he clearly chair bound or bed bound and dependent on someone else for all ADLS/IADLs?

Much of what the OASIS is looking for is common sense answers about the patient's ability at this very moment. Don't anticipate or read into the questions.

After you have done a few of these, you may find you are actually able to complete much of the form after your visit by closing your eyes and replaying the visit in your mind.

The SOC OASIS data points for Clinical, Functional and Social information are transmitted to CMS along with the ICD codes for diagnoses pertaining to the care to be provided. This signals to CMS that an episode of care has begun. An algorithm is generated and a CASE MIX code produced. This CASE MIX code determines the PPS (prospective pay) allowed for that episode. So your answers to OASIS questions are vital to the reimbursement rate for this patient's care in this episode.

This lump sum payment will cover all costs related to the care for this 60-day episode. You will have to work with your administration to determine the budget for the number of visits for each discipline and incidentals such as supplies. From this the 485, your plan of care, is derived with specific MD orders unique to this patient. It includes goals and end points for all disciplines. The MD must sign it in a timely manner for your agency to be able to bill for the episode.

During the episode of care there are points at which the Therapist (if one has been ordered) must report progress and measurable gains as well as goals for continued care to CMS. Once again the time frame and actual content of these reports has and will continue to change to meet the needs and requirements for CMS. Consult your administrative staff for guidance.

RECERTIFICATION OASIS

At the end of the 60-day episode, if the patient still meets criteria for skilled care, a **Recertification OASIS** form is completed by the primary case manager which can be either the RN or Therapist. The form itself is usually filled out about 7-10 days prior to the end of the episode. Your agency will have a process for this and usually the case is presented at Case Conference to determine the eligibility in advance of the Recert.

Submitting the data to CMS signals the care continues and another 60-day episode has begun. Forms to update orders and POC (485) as well as an order to recertify the patient with the new episode dates on it may also be required.

Again the OASIS data in this form along with the ICD codes generate the CASE MIX code that determines the reimbursement for this 60-day episode.

TRANSFER OASIS

If the patient is hospitalized or moves to a skilled nursing facility during the episode, you complete the **Transfer OASIS** form and it is submitted to CMS. This signals the patient has been put on hold in anticipation of a return.

Your agency will probably require some additional paperwork and procedure such as:

- an MD order to place visits "on hold" due to transfer / hospitalization
- a call to the discharge planner at the facility to notify them the patient is on care with your agency
- scheduled phone calls to track the hospitalization and ensure the patient is returned to your agency for care
- remind caregivers or family to call your agency when the patient is expected to be discharged home and have the facility refer back to your agency

If the patient has no intention of returning, the **Transfer/ Discharge box** is checked and no further OASIS data is needed. Once submitted to CMS, the status becomes Discharged and the episode is ended as of that date. Notification of the physician and an order to discharge will be in order.

RESUMPTION OASIS

If the patient is discharged back home, you will complete the **Resumption OASIS** form to establish and report changes in primary diagnosis, skilled need and clinical issues, functional status, and social issues. Again you will assess for skilled need, homebound status and establish a new POC with the patient and physician. If the primary diagnosis changes, the reimbursement may be adjusted.

DISCHARGE OASIS

Once the patient meets all measurable goals, or plateaus and is unable to progress any further, the skilled need ends and the patient must be discharged. Hopefully you have prepared the patient and family for this day and he is ready to assume full responsibility for his own care and health status. (Remember discharge planning BEGINS at SOC.) The skilled discipline making the last visit of the episode will complete the Discharge OASIS which is not as complex as the SOC form, but demonstrates the outcomes which are hopefully positive. Any other agency required forms such as an MD order to discharge would be filled out as well.

A few last notes about the OASIS process:

I have heard nurses say the OASIS process is a classic application of the Nursing Process in which we assess and evaluate, plan care, implement the care and evaluate the outcomes. For nurses, it actually helps you provide <u>pure nursing care</u>.

The OASIS is a tool that lets us evaluate and demonstrate the quality of care the professional staff provides. It benchmarks your agency against others to provide consumers an option for informed choice for the best possible outcomes based on their needs.

The OASIS requires critical thinking and focused attention to detail. It's a necessary evil, but if you sit back and evaluate the document, it will help you assess the patient's needs and establish measurable goals to improve your patient's outcomes and health status.

<u>Note:</u> One situation that seems to happen often is a Recert is due at the same time you Resume a patient and yes, you will have to compete BOTH OASIS forms and all accompanying items your agency requires in order to continue the care, generate the CASE MIX code and be able to bill for the episode.

WHAT IS a LUPA?

The premise of the 60-day episode is that a patient will require a minimum of 5 visits to provide the care and meet the established goals. If 4 or fewer visits are made, it does not constitute an episode and becomes a **LUPA (Low Utilization Payment Adjustment)**. These visits are then paid as fee-for service. They are somewhat frowned upon by CMS and should be minimized whenever possible.

In many instances, the LUPA can be avoided by assessing the patient's needs and anticipating future needs to help prevent accidents, recurrent illness, and complication from chronic illness In essence reducing the need for future hospitalizations as well.

Consider the patient may need at least 2 Skilled Nurse visits to ensure he understands and is following directions for medications, diet and other treatment modalities such as oxygen, nebulizers, inhalers, etc.

At least 1 PT visit for home safety evaluation and fall prevention. Instruction such as Caregiver training in body mechanics, transfer training, and proper use of DME are other things to consider for PT participation. Perhaps 2 or more visits would be indicated.

An OT can help with assessing for grab bars and where to place them, teaching ADL assistance such as bathing, grooming, feeding techniques for caregivers, or assessing for devices and changes for the patient to remain independent in his ADLs. Energy conservation training is often overlooked and is an important component for cardiac and pulmonary patients as well as anyone recovering from an acute illness, surgery or injury.

One or two visits from a HHA to instruct the family or caregivers in how to safely and efficiently bathe, shower and shampoo the patient can also be very beneficial.

And finally the MSW can provide valuable community resources for short term and long term planning along with counseling and active listening for coping with lifestyle changes both temporary and permanent.

If you make any combination of 5 or more visits from these disciplines, you will have completed your 5 visit requirement to establish an episode and avoid the LUPA. Remember however, the POC must be unique to the needs of the individual patient and you should not establish a routine of plans of care that are exactly alike for all your patients. Just keep this scenario of needs in mind and apply to patients as needed.

WHAT is an OUTLIER?

Another term you will hear is **OUTLIER**. The general philosophy of home health care is to get in, teach the patient or caregiver, and get out (discharge). Like anything else, there are the exceptions to this "rule". You will encounter some patients who require ongoing frequent visits for care such as complicated, slow healing wounds, or diabetic care and daily insulin administration where no other solution exists.

These OUTLIER episodes create costs that exceed the standard PPS payment schedule and consequently will be paid on an adjusted schedule. Agencies cannot refuse to admit patients who present the possibility of becoming outliers and cannot discharge until other arrangements are made. However, everyone strives to find solutions as quickly as possible and help patients and caregivers assume care and responsibility to reduce the number of OUTLIERS on service.

CHAPTER EIGHT: A Few Loose Ends

I hope that I have given you enough insight to help you decide to make the transition and to understand your new role. If you enjoy one-on-one patient interaction, educating patients, and helping them to remain in their own homes and as independent as possible you will come to love being part of the home health care realm.

Be prepared to make an investment in your own equipment. Keep your receipts because in most cases this is a tax deduction. You'll need bag to carry your basic equipment such as stethoscope, sphygmomanometer, thermometer (a digital tympanic is a good choice), bandage scissors, calipers, gate belt, gloves, hand sanitizer, etc. Some items might be furnished by your agency such as the hand sanitizer and gloves, but most of the other items you will likely have to purchase.

For your own safety and infection control you should have clothing and shoes that you only wear for work.

Keep receipts and records for your purchases, your gasoline usage, mileage for work and expenses related to your car and your phone. Some or all of it can be tax deductible. Consult with your tax advisor for specific instructions.

One of the things that can be very hard to do is to <u>let go of some of the control</u> you have in other settings. This can be especially challenging for ICU nurses who have so much responsibility for their patients. They make some of the very best home health nurses because their knowledge and experience base is vast and they are used to using their critical thinking skills and making decisions on the fly. They often develop strong rapports with the MDs for their assessment skills and ability to make suggestions.

However, in my experience these nurses also have the most difficult time with letting the patient learn to take responsibility for their own care. When your patient is at home with an IV on a pump, you have to be able to sleep at night and not worry that it will infiltrate or run dry because you aren't there.

You have to teach them what to do and what to watch for and allow them to be responsible.

You also need to be able to walk in to a new admission and figure out what his skilled and other needs are without being given a task list to follow. *Much of what we do in home health care is not task oriented.* Associated perhaps, but not always the driving force. Patient education is a broad term and figuring out *what they don't know that they don't know* can be complicated.

For example, never assume a patient understands his medications just because he's been taking them for years. Ask what he knows and you'll most likely be surprised. And when they compare notes with their friends-- watch out! And the ways people spice up a no-salt diet can be flabbergasting! Along with the incredibly unsafe practices they implement in their homes. And throw rugs on top of throw rugs along with piles of newspapers everywhere…and they know if you take any away!

There will never be a dull day in home health care. You will learn things you never knew you needed to know and you'll meet some of the most fascinating people in the world. Some you will want to take home with you and others you can't discharge fast enough! Enjoy the experience!

Some Suggested Resources

Tina M. Marrelli MSN MA RN. *Handbook of Home Health Standards - Revised Reprint: Quality, Documentation, and Reimbursement, 5e (Handbook of Home Health Standards & Documentation Guidelines for Reimbursement)* Spiral-bound – Mosby; July 14, 2011. [A new edition is available from her website: www.marelli.com]

Karen McGough Monks MSN, RN. *Pocket Guide to Home Health Care.* Spiral bound- W.B. Saunders Company; 2000.

Melinda Gaboury, COS-C. *Pocket Guide to OASIS-C1.* HCPro; spi edition 2015.

Home Health Quality Initiative
https://www.cms.gov/Medicare/Quality-Initiatives-Patient-Assessment-Instruments/HomeHealthQualityInits/index.html

Medicare Learning Network : The Medicare Home Health Benefit https://www.cms.gov/Outreach-and-Education/Medicare-Learning-Network-MLN/MLNProducts/Downloads/Home-Health-Benefit-Fact-Sheet-ICN908143.pdf

American Association of Home Care

https://www.aahomecare.org/

National Association of Home Care & Hospice

http://www.nahc.org/

Visiting Nurses of America   http://www.vnaa.org/

Home Health Compare   https://www.medicare.gov/
homehealthcompare/

OASIS   https://www.cms.gov/Medicare/Quality-Initiatives-
Patient-Assessment-Instruments/OASIS/index.html

More resources are listed on my websites:

HomeHealth101.com

Housecalls-Online.com

CONTACT ME:

If you wish to use any of this copyrighted material, please
contact me for written permission, details, and costs.

Homehealthnurse727@gmail.com.

About Kathy Quan

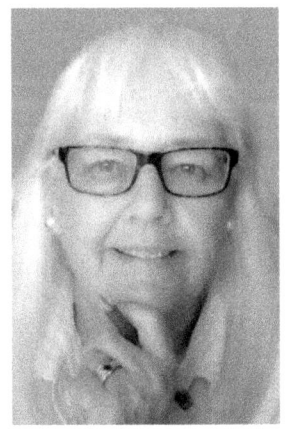

Kathy Quan RN BSN PHN has been a nurse for over thirty-five years. The majority of her career has been in home health and hospice. She has been a field nurse, nursing supervisor, acting branch manager and QAPI specialist. Today she works part time for hospice as a QAPI specialist.

Kathy is an award-winning author of six books including *The Everything Guide to Caring for Aging Parents*, which is based on her experience as a home health nurse and administrator. In 2004, Kathy became the last Guide to Nursing at About.com and has written for many other nursing and health care sites. She has several blogs and websites.

In 1997, she started a website for home health nurses, Housecalls-Online.com and a few years later added HomeHealth101.com to her repertoire of websites and blogs. Both of these sites are meant to be an extension of her passion and quest to mentor new staff to the home health care field. Improving documentation is an on going learning process, and Kathy loves to be a part of it.

Kathy has also taught classes in:
- how to care for your aging parents
- how to find a career in health care,
- Home Health Documentation

Recently Kathy has participated in several Google Hangouts and other web-based podcasts and webinars for nurses and the healthcare community on such topics as collaborating in social media, and how to renew your love and passion for nursing.

More about Kathy at KathyQuan.com

BOOKS BY KATHY QUAN
- *The Everything New Nurse Book*, 2006; Adams Media
- *The Everything Guide to Health Care Careers*, 2006; Adams Media
- *150 Tips and Tricks for New Nurses*, 2009; Adams Media
- *The Everything Guide to Caring for Aging Parents*, 2009; Adams Media
- *The Everything New Nurse Book, 2nd Edition*, 2011; Adams Media
- *The New Nurse Handbook*, 2014; Fall River Press
- *Exploring the Home Health Care Experience*, 2015; Kathy Quan publisher

Kathy has also contributed to multiple other publications. You can find a list of these at KathyQuan.com